THY
CINE
RISH

C000260628

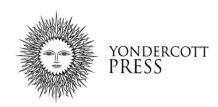

YONDERCOTT PRESS

Published in the UK by Yondercott Press
an imprint of Alternative Training Limited
Orchard Leigh · Rodborough Hill
Stroud · Gloucestershire · GL5 3SS

First published: 2007
Website: www.yondercottpress.com
Email: info@yondercottpress.com
© Yondercott Press

ISBN: 978-0-9544766-1-8

Printed and bound in the UK by Lotus Design & Print
Written by Mo Morrish
Edited by Delny Britton
Design and typesetting by Mani Norland

British Library Cataloguing in Publishing Data. A catalogue
record for this book is available from the British Library.

EDITOR'S NOTE

We have chosen to use the 'oeo' spelling of homoeopathy as it is closer to the original Greek. When referencing we have deferred to the individual authors who have chosen to use the more modern and Americanised 'eo' spelling i.e. homeopathy.

DEDICATION

To each and every person I have met
in homoeopathic consultation I offer
a heartfelt 'thank you'. It has been
an enormous privilege and I have
learnt so much from you. I hope I
can pass on what you have taught
me for the benefit of others.

CONTENTS

ACKNOWLEDGEMENTS

HOMOEOPATHY : A RATIONAL CHOICE IN MEDICINE

ACKNOWLEDGEMENTS

A special thank you to Ruth Sewell for her foreword and for her strong suggestion that I get this book written!

To my team of colleagues, friends and patients who have read rough drafts, found references and offered advice and encouragement: thank you. You include Elaine Watson, Lisa Mansell, Debbie Schofield, Anthony Bickley, Sarah Bickley, Ian Webster, Sarah Hayden-Binder, Wayne Allen, Ali Pennicott and Carol Boyce.

Huge thanks to Delny Britton for solid and insightful input on all levels, skilful editing and helping me to keep the edge. Warm thanks also to Mani Norland for encouragement, sass and getting it out there!

Lastly, a special thanks to my wife Ali for the sharing of our homoeopathic practice and the enjoyment of seeing so many people get themselves better.

FOREWORD

I am delighted to have been asked to write the foreword to Mo's book. I have known Mo for many years and greatly admire his personal qualities of straightforwardness and gentleness of heart. He is a highly experienced homoeopath with a strong commitment to integrated and holistic medicine and the education of homoeopathic practitioners. I know his patients benefit greatly from his healing art; I also know that as a skilled and insightful teacher he makes an enormous contribution not only to individual students but also to the wider field of homoeopathic medicine at this time.

Along with other colleagues in mainstream healthcare and complementary medicine I am concerned at the increasing trend in some circles to malign homoeopathy and only present evidence that suggests 'homoeopathy doesn't work'. As a patient of homoeopathy, and especially as a psychotherapist who has confidently referred clients to homoeopaths for over 20 years, I have experienced myself and witnessed in others the gentle and decisive ability of an accurately prescribed homoeopathic remedy to initiate a healing response. Homoeopathy is capable of helping the patient by seeing them as a whole person and not just a collection of symptoms to be controlled. It gets to the heart of what disturbs the patient's life and state of health and invites them to be involved in their own healing process. It has the amazing potential to facilitate a return to personal levels of balanced health and wellbeing.

I am in no doubt that homoeopathy is a potent and highly relevant form of medicine. It can be used as a single source of support and it can also work in an integrated way with other approaches. The most important thing for me is to encourage you to open your mind, to read this book and to make your own decisions.

Ruth Sewell PhD
Lecturer in Integrated Cancer Care and Psychotherapist.

INTRODUCTION

You may be curious about homoeopathy or be in the process of deciding whether or not to consult a homoeopath. You may be confused because what you have read about homoeopathy in the national press is at odds with what you hear from people who have actually tried homoeopathy.

You may be one of those satisfied people, delighted with your homoeopathic treatment yet wanting to know more about it.

This has been written for you.

Much of what is written about homoeopathy in journals, newspapers and websites is negative and attacking. Most of the people who write these articles know very little about homoeopathy. Much of what is written, therefore, is not true.

This book has been written to put that right, to bring perspective, to give you the chance to make an informed choice. The simple fact is that homoeopathic medicine works well enough and often enough for millions of people to use it to help them recover from injury and disease. We have found something here. We have a resource to help us to heal ourselves and become truly well. And we squabble over it!

Meanwhile more and more of us are suffering from an ever-increasing range of health problems and our health services are not coping. In this book I suggest that suffering people are not served by squabbling and that the only sane and sensible solution is to find a way of working together, of integrating different medical approaches.

You do not have to agree with everything written here, I only hope that you may be stimulated to become more informed. I also hope that you may feel empowered to re-take responsibility for what is arguably the most important aspect of your life...your health and that of your family.

I have chosen to write simply of sometimes complex matters and to include a comprehensive list of resources for those of you who may wish to explore further.

I hope this will be helpful to you.

CLEARING THE WAY

Homoeopathy is an important and long-established system of medicine. It is a beautiful synthesis of science, philosophy and experience into a medical art whose practise is both simple and profound. Almost any condition that you might take to a GP would benefit from the homoeopathic approach, as millions of people will testify. Strangely, scorn and derision is poured upon it regularly from the great, and seemingly illustrious height of medical orthodoxy. It is frequently written that 'homoeopathy does not work', that it is 'unscientific', that its practitioners are all 'quacks' and that it amounts to 'nothing more than water'. Most of the detractors claim to be scientists, as if that also makes them good ones. Most of them know very little about homoeopathy.

Many people are sceptical about homoeopathy. It is entirely reasonable to be sceptical but it is not reasonable to be dogmatic. Orthodox scientific thinking tells us that the idea of homoeopathy is absurd: cutting edge scientific thinking suggests that homoeopathy is not nearly as absurd as we thought. The 'new physics' (now nearly 100 years old) and recent research into the previously unknown properties of water (1) as well as the relatively new science of psychoneuroimmunology are beginning to reveal an increasingly subtle world of energy and the inter-connectedness of all things. In this new understanding homoeopathy begins to make scientific sense.

There is a general and unspoken assumption that everything that homoeopathy supposedly is not (effective, scientific, safe, proven) modern mainstream medicine is. It is not in our best interest to continue with this assumption because, as we shall see later, it is simply not true.

Mainstream medicine might be so named because in Western culture particularly, and at this time, it is the most believed in, most life-saving (not the same as life-enhancing) and best-advertised medical practice. This has not always been the case. In Western culture before the accidental 'discovery' of penicillin, doctors were not afforded the respect and prestige they have been since. Meanwhile in other cultures, China and India for example, traditional systems of medicine have been helping to restore and maintain health for thousands of years.

It is interesting that modern mainstream medicine seems to have appropriated the terms 'medical' and 'medicine' for itself. Phrases such as 'from a medical point of view' and 'medical training', suggest that there is only one system of medicine on Earth. Might there not be some arrogance here?

There are, in fact, many medical points of view and many kinds of medical training, for example: Ayurvedic, herbal, traditional Chinese, osteopathic, naturopathic, anthroposophical, homoeopathic or modern mainstream.

What I find alarming about modern mainstream medicine is that there are no principles upon which it is based. A principle is an underlying guiding theory, a basic tenet, and a fundamental truth. There is no fundamental truth in mainstream medicine. Theories constantly change, 'wonder drugs' appear and disappear and, until the very recent drive for evidence-based medicine, practitioners based their work only upon opinion.

Let me be clear that I have immense respect and admiration for doctors, nurses and frontline healthcare workers. I have immense respect and admiration for much of what mainstream medicine has achieved. What I want to do is to put it in perspective, to be clear that it is extremely helpful in many healthcare situations and not at all in others.

I would like us to respect all useful systems of medicine and have them available to us all. I would like all health service users to be able to consult with as wide a range of medical practitioners as possible so that we can all make well-informed decisions about our health. This is called an integrated approach to medicine. It involves all of us growing up, thinking for ourselves, taking responsibility for our health and respecting different ways of practising the high art of medicine.

I understand that this maturity will not come about easily.

MEDICINE

The word medicine comes from the word mederi; it means 'to heal'. To heal means to restore to health, to make whole again. Healing, curing, restoring is a process through which a diseased patient returns to health. This process happens naturally (called recovery) or is stimulated by an agent, treatment or action.

I know of no agent, treatment or action particular to mainstream medicine that heals. Not one. The antibiotic, for example, is said to cure infectious diseases such as pneumonia. This is not true. When it 'works', which is not always, the antibiotic only kills the invading bacteria: it does not stimulate the patient to heal; at most it buys a breathing space for recovery to take place naturally. Even surgery, which can be fantastic in bringing shattered bodies back together, can only create the opportunity within which that body can heal itself.

The body has a well-known and amazing capacity to heal itself. Doctors rely upon this 'body wisdom' to enable patients to recover after surgery or other acute interventions. And wouldn't it be both exciting and sensible to study the mechanisms of the spontaneous remission of cancers and other seemingly 'incurable' diseases? These self-healings happen so why don't we research them more? The reason is likely to be that there is no money to be made.

Thus there is nothing medicinal in mainstream medicine. It does not use medicines or treatments to stimulate or encourage healing. Instead, it uses drugs and treatments to alleviate, control and suppress symptoms. This is, of course, extremely useful in certain situations but it is not to be confused with real medicine.

Homoeopathic medicine, on the other hand, uses micro-doses of substances to stimulate and encourage the individual patient to return to health. Thus it is a true system of medicine.

MAINSTREAM MEDICINE

Modern mainstream medicine, without doubt, provides the best emergency treatment service on Earth. Daily, in emergency rooms everywhere, people are saved from death. In the wake of terrorism, war and natural disaster modern medicine preserves life on a scale so awesome that it can seem miraculous. Millions of lives are saved every year.

In the treatment of chronic diseases such as arthritis, asthma, cancer etc. and psychological diseases, the situation is considerably less positive. Chronic diseases are not decreasing; they are increasing, despite billions of pounds spent and extraordinary effort made.

Another kind of disease is also on the increase: iatrogenic disease. Iatros means 'doctor' and iatrogenic diseases are those caused by doctors and their treatments. Every year hundreds of thousands of people have their health undermined or destroyed by drugs and treatments prescribed by doctors everywhere. A British Medical Association report has estimated that more than 250,000 patients are admitted to hospital every year in the United Kingdom because of harmful effects after taking prescribed drugs (2). Obviously this is not intentional, nonetheless it is a fact and it adds to the suffering.

Modern mainstream medicine is always described as being 'scientific'. What does this mean, and how scientific is it in reality? Science comes from the Latin word, *scientia*, which means knowledge. Knowledge is gained through the 'systematic study of the nature and behaviour of the material and physical universe' (Collins dictionary). This study is based upon 'observation, experiment and measurement and leads to the formulation of laws to describe these facts in general terms.'

This standard definition suggests a certain bias for the material as opposed to the non-material aspects of the universe such as energy, consciousness, emotion or life itself. Since the 'new physics' of Einstein and others confirms that everything is essentially energy in some form, I offer a slight modification to the definition of science: 'The systematic study of the nature and behaviour of the material and non-material universe etc.'

For such observation/experiment to be valid it needs to be unprejudiced, that is with no element of pre-judgement. In this way things are observed more as they are and less as the observer influences them to be.

From studies in quantum physics we now understand that the observer participates in the observation, interacts with what is being observed. As objective as we try to be we cannot help but bring our subjective selves to the observation/experiment: the researcher is part of the research. If we are simply exploring then we find what we find. If we are biased by an intention to find something particular, to prove or dis-prove something, then we are more likely to find what we are looking for. Totally unprejudiced observation is impossible yet it is something to which all true scientists aspire.

Measurement too has limitation. We cannot measure life, mind or emotion yet this does not mean that they do not exist. Size, degree and quantity are available to be measured but quality is not. We can measure many aspects of a dolphin, but we cannot measure dolphin as a whole, we cannot measure the essence of dolphin. We cannot measure the essence of a disease such as influenza. And we cannot measure emotions such as anger, grief or love.

Mainstream medicine could be said to be scientific in as much as it is based upon observation, experiment and measurement. However, it is very difficult to say how unprejudiced the observers, experimenters and measurers might be. Given that the majority of them are influenced by the pharmaceutical industry in terms of research grants, salaries and other benefits, bias is likely to have a significant financial advantage. Given also that the industry is self-regulating, any bias is likely to be well protected!

As I understand it no law has been formulated to describe mainstream medicine in general terms. The one law that was formulated was then abandoned. With regard to the effect of medicines on sick people, the Arndt-Schultz Law maintains that: small doses stimulate, medium doses paralyse and large doses kill. This echoes the homoeopathic principle of the minimum dose yet was abandoned by orthodox pharmacy because 'small/medium/large' are imprecise terms (and because there is no money to be made from 'small doses'?). They are by nature relative to one another and relate to the individuality of the patient. This is not regarded as important within mainstream medicine.

The working model upon which mainstream medicine is based is materialistic and molecular and informed chiefly by Newtonian, rather than modern quantum, physics (Newton died in 1727). It is a useful model that regards the patient as a fantastic and self-regulating machine largely controlled and directed by a kind of supercomputer, the brain. As useful as this model might be, it is out of date. It is not informed by cutting-edge science, by research that confirms the universe to be essentially non-material and non-mechanical (3).

Much of the study of mainstream medicine has centred around the dissection and examination of dead humans. Dead humans are noticeably different to ones that are alive and this focus may have contributed to the de-humanisation of mainstream medicine. (Not before time, young doctors are now being trained to have more awareness of the person inside 'the machine'.)

Disease is regarded as impairment in the normal functioning of the machine and drugs and treatments are directed to the parts affected. These drugs and treatments are prescribed to have a particular action with little or no consideration for any other actions or effects within the patient. An antibiotic, for example, may be prescribed for an infection in the right ear yet it is obvious that molecules of the drug will travel throughout the body and have other, not always beneficial, effects elsewhere. If a number of parts are affected then a number of drugs or treatments may be prescribed. There appears to be no real acknowledgement that all parts are connected and that a change induced in one part might affect another part or, indeed, the whole.

Many people end up being prescribed an increasing number of different drugs with inadequate monitoring and no possibility of knowing their combined effects. Often a single drug or a combination of drugs will induce new symptoms. These are called 'side-effects' or 'adverse drug reactions' (ADR) and can range from itching and vomiting to psychotic behaviour (and in extreme cases, death). Further drugs and treatments may be introduced to counter these effects and so it becomes impossible to know what drug is having what effect, harmful or beneficial. This is ill logic; it is not good science.

It is generally accepted that adverse drug reactions are under-reported and accurate figures are difficult to obtain, but it would seem that up to 40% of people experience side effects when taking prescribed drugs and a significant number of these are fatal (4). Hospitals, too, are dangerous places in which, every year, thousands of patients develop life-threatening illnesses (such as infection with MRSA), are left with a severe disability or die as a direct consequence of being admitted. Hundreds of thousands of people are more ill when they come out of hospital than when they go in (5). In America, the total number of deaths in one year alone caused by conventional medicine was an astounding 783,936 (6). This figure is the equivalent of six jumbo jet planes falling out of the sky every day! It has become evident that 'government approved medicine' is now the leading cause of death and injury in the US.

Mainstream medicine saves life…it also kills, maims and undermines health. People in Western cultures might live longer than they used to but their quality of health is not improving.

In addition, modern mainstream medicine is not nearly as scientific as we have been lead to believe. To continue to insist that mainstream medicine is the best and most scientific system of medicine on Earth seems both patronising and insulting to human intelligence.

HOMOEOPATHY

Homoeopathy is a rational system of medicine based upon principles that are easy to understand (see 'Principles') and follow the laws of nature. Homoeopathy is not a belief system or part of any religion. It is not an alternative to modern mainstream medicine. No single system of medicine can reasonably claim to have a monopoly on healing - we need all the help we can get!

There are circumstances in which many experienced holistic medical practitioners consider homoeopathy to be particularly useful:

1 In the treatment of shock and trauma, mental, emotional or physical, and any health problems consequent to them.
2 In the treatment of health problems consequent to infectious disease, surgery, vaccination, anaesthesia and chemotherapy or other poisonings.
3 In the promotion of health on all levels - mental, emotional, spiritual and physical (this is known as 'constitutional treatment', see later).

There are circumstances when mainstream medicine would be the first choice of many holistic medical practitioners:

1 In life-threatening situations.
2 In situations where surgical intervention is necessary.

There are circumstances when homoeopathy and mainstream medicine work well together in an integrated manner. Palliative care and recovery from trauma and surgery are the most commonly encountered examples.

Homoeopathy takes nothing away from the mainstream medical model; it simply takes notice of something that is always present in a live person. Life force, vital force or 'bio' force is the force or energy that enlivens or animates the body of living beings. It is an instinctual force that moves molecules, maintains harmonious structure and function, organises the healing of wounds and leaves at the time of death. If you have ever seen a dead body or been with someone when they died you will know what I am talking about. An adult human is composed of billions of cells, trillions of atoms, and is constantly re-composing itself in the course of a life. After death, once this animating force has left, the body decomposes.

Thus this life/bio force somehow organises molecules into a highly complex living organism and facilitates the constant flow of information between all parts. We cannot see or measure this force any more than we can see or measure life itself, we can only observe the phenomena that it produces, yet to simply ignore it seems absurd.

From a single double-stranded molecule of DNA to the end of a long life, the human organism exists and experiences itself at many different levels, simultaneously. In health, mental, emotional and physical aspects of being are harmoniously coordinated. This involves a quite extraordinary degree of energetic, chemical and neural communication between the body and the mind.

The homoeopathic medical model has, for over 200 years, placed great emphasis on the unity of the mind and body and the importance of mental and emotional symptoms in patients. Now the relatively new science of psychoneuroimmunology (which studies the effects of thinking and feeling upon the body) reveals, beyond any doubt, that psyche (non-material aspects such as mind and emotions) is directly linked to, and forms an information network with, soma (material aspects such as molecules and organs). In mainstream medicine the term 'psychosomatic illness' has had a very negative connotation and the role of emotions in the cause and treatment of disease has generally been disregarded. There is now overwhelming evidence that this approach is incorrect. Put simply, what we think and feel affects our body chemistry and hence our health: mind and matter are intimately connected (7). Psychoneuroimmunology supports homoeopathic thinking and is contributing to the 're-humanising' of medicine.

The word health comes from 'hale', meaning 'whole'. From this we can arrive at 'holism' or the holistic perspective: seeing the wholeness in things. Mainstream medical thinking is not holistic. It is predominantly left-brained and analytical, reducing everything to its component parts. In practice this often means that a patient may be under the care of a number of consultants with no one person looking after him/her as a whole person.

Homoeopathy insists upon both left- (logical, analytical) and right-brain (bringing things together, seeing patterns in complexity) activity, and on viewing the mind and body as one inter-connected whole. In this way it is more 'whole brained', holistic and healthy in its approach to healing.

Health, from the homoeopathic perspective, is seen as a state of relative ease and freedom. This occurs when the whole person is functioning harmoniously on all levels, physical, mental and emotional, and is fulfilling him or herself socially and spiritually. The life force is flowing in order and all is well. Disease is seen as a disturbance in the flow of life force. The organism is stressed/distressed and this results in disturbance in normal sensation and function, experienced as symptoms.

In this way disease is regarded as a dynamic disturbance of the whole person. Symptoms may be produced anywhere within the body-mind yet the whole organism is diseased, not just a part. As an example, cancer is a disease of the whole person and the tumour is a local expression of that.

All symptoms on all levels, mental, emotional and physical, are considered and evaluated by a homoeopath. Those that are most characteristic of and particular to the patient are the ones most useful to the homoeopath in the process of selecting the best homoeopathic medicine.

Example 1: A man in a hospital ward suffering with pneumonia. He lies very still with his back to everyone and periodically sits up to drink an entire glass of cold water. Groaning, he lies back down again and when the nurse asks if he is alright he curtly tells her to leave him alone.

Example 2: Another man in a hospital bed suffering with pneumonia. He is sitting up in bed with three pillows and sipping from a glass of cold water. He is well groomed, wears an immaculate silk dressing gown and holds onto the nurse's hand because he does not want to be left alone.

Both men are suffering with pneumonia and both men have been prescribed the same antibiotic which may or may not be helpful. Can you see that they are in different disease states and so need different medicines? They are each expressing 'pneumonia' in their own individual way.

The homoeopath always wonders what is causing a symptom, what is behind it, what is it expressing? To numb, remove or suppress symptoms without attempting to address the underlying cause is to deny any possibility of cure and is not good science. It is also potentially very dangerous. Imagine that you are driving and a warning light flashes on your car dashboard: how would you feel if the mechanic simply stuck some tape over it or removed the bulb?

Individuality is at the core of homoeopathic thinking. That every human being is unique is a fact of genetics. Every human being reacts to environment and circumstances in an individual way; every human being lives his or her life in an individual way; every human being suffers and dies in an individual way. Whilst we obviously have so much in common, we all have our own unique way of being in the world, our own 'bio-story'.

It is impossible to predict with certainty how any one person will react to a virus, drug, medicine, vaccine, food etc. What is certain is that some people react very negatively and may even die, whilst others survive and even grow stronger through the experience. These things are individual and relate to the susceptibility of the person.

Homoeopathy seeks to understand the unique way in which every person creates and expresses his or her disease. Each person is offered an individual prescription and treatment plan. The optimum dose of medicine for each individual is discovered (because it cannot be known any other way) by starting treatment with a minimum dose and observing the effects. This is rational, obvious and good science.

Homoeopathic medicine is based upon observation, experiment and measurement and is organised in a systematic manner (See: 'Provings' later). The homoeopathic observers, experimenters and measurers are not likely to be prejudiced as there is no advantage to be gained. In fact in homoeopathy, prejudice prejudices a positive outcome! The principles of symptom similarity, minimum dose, single medicine etc. (see 'Principles') have been formulated to describe homoeopathy in general terms and the obvious conclusion is that homoeopathy is a scientific system of medicine, much more so than its mainstream equivalent.

THE PRINCIPLES

'The highest ideal of cure is the rapid, gentle and permanent
restoration of health; that is the lifting and annihilation
of the disease in its entire extent in the shortest, most
reliable and least disadvantageous way, according to
clearly realisable principles.'

Dr. S. Hahnemann, Founder of Homoeopathy

One of the strengths of homoeopathic medicine is that it is based upon
principles. This is not the case with mainstream medicine. At any time
in the future (and on any other planet!) homoeopathy will be practised
in the same way as it is now: if it is not then it will not be homoeopathy.
There are no latest theories, no new wonder drugs, just an ongoing
refinement of a system that has already proved itself to the satisfaction
of patients and practitioners alike. As a practitioner I find this reassuring
when caught up in the often-complex process of helping people return
to health. What follows is a simplified and distilled description of the
essential principles.

Symptom Similarity

Homoeopathy means 'similar suffering'. Natural substances (plants,
minerals etc.) that can cause symptoms in a healthy person can be used
to cure similar symptoms in a person who is ill. Hippocrates, the father
of Western medicine, discussed healing with similars over two thousand
years ago. This approach, often expressed as 'like cures like', is based
on a simple observation that has been verified over and over in the
successful treatment of millions of people around the world.

Example: have you ever smoked a cigarette? Many people have described their first experience of this as 'horrible':

'My heart started racing and I suddenly felt icy cold and deathly sick. I retched a few times and then threw up. I was shivering by this time and my mouth had gone from really dry to being full of saliva that I wanted to spit out. I felt better sitting down outside but when I smelt the cigarette smoke I wanted to throw up again.'

This scenario is often observed on cross-channel ferries and the homoeopathic medicine Tabacum, made from tobacco, has a good reputation in helping people who are suffering from travel sickness.

Provings
A proving (from the German, pruefung, meaning 'test') is the process through which the potential medicinal uses of a natural substance are discovered. Healthy human volunteers undergo a full homoeopathic consultation and their current state of health is evaluated. They then participate in a double blind, placebo-controlled randomised experiment in which the substance being tested is administered. No participant has any idea what is being tested or whether he or she has taken it or placebo.

The 'provers' then carefully record all changes in their health, all changes in normal sensation and function. This includes any dreams of note, any moods, perceptions or persistent thoughts. Every day the prover speaks with an individually assigned supervisor whose task is to help clarify the information. Only when symptoms cease is the proving over for that individual and, following a final conversation with the supervisor, the prover's journal is handed in to the proving coordinator. Collating all the information gathered in all the provers' journals and then arranging it systematically is a long and painstaking task. Nonetheless, the health of a patient may one day depend upon such accurate observation and recording.

All this information is then organised into the homoeopathic Materia Medica. This consists of detailed information on over 3000 medicines. To help find the correct medicine, information on symptoms - and which medicinal substance causes them - is organised into what is known as a Homoeopathic Clinical Repertory. This is a kind of guidebook or index to the Materia Medica.

Proving accounts and the Materia Medica provide a vast store of medical knowledge and the homoeopath spends a huge amount of time and energy studying them. The matching of patient symptoms to proving symptoms involves a methodical process that is part of the science of homoeopathy.

Potencies

Homoeopathic medicines are prescribed in a specially prepared form: the potency. To avoid the potential poisoning effects of a medicinal substance, whilst maintaining its curative effects, it is subjected to a process of repeated dilution and succussion. Succussion means that after each serial dilution the medicine is exposed to a vigorous shaking. It is not understood what happens during this process but it appears that succussion allows the medicinal power of the substance to be enhanced well beyond what is possible with simple dilution. This process diminishes the negative effects of the crude medicinal substance yet harnesses and increases its potential to cure. Hence 'potency'.

Most homoeopathic medicines are prepared using the centesimal scale of potency and dilution. By this I mean that a single drop of a solution of the material substance is diluted in 99 drops of alcohol. This is 1c. Diluting one drop of a 1c solution in 99 drops of alcohol gives us a 2c, and so on. There is no limit to this process. Once past the 12th dilution orthodox science tells us that there will be no molecules of the original substance left in solution. Homoeopaths commonly prescribe potencies of 30c and higher.

Mainstream medical thought requires that a drug has an 'active ingredient'. This has obvious importance if the medical model is molecular and material. The homoeopathic medical model includes the intangible life force, is both molecular and non-material, and so 'molecules of active ingredient' are much less relevant.

That potencies have a curative effect has been observed for centuries (see 'Evidence'). How a potency affects a patient is still unknown.

Science does not have answers to everything, yet I have every confidence that good science will explain this phenomenon in time, if given a chance. We need to direct research into finding out more.

'One thing I have learned in a long life: that all our science, measured against reality, is primitive and childlike - and yet it is the most precious thing we have.'

Albert Einstein

The Single Medicine and Minimum Dose

Homoeopathic medicines stimulate the natural healing processes of each individual patient. In this way the patient restores him/herself to health. The least degree of medicinal stimulus necessary to induce a curative response is the ideal. Obviously. If only one medicine or drug is prescribed at any one time then it is reasonable to ascribe any subsequent effects to it. If more than one medicine or drug is prescribed at any one time it is impossible to be sure what is having what effect.

Homoeopaths prescribe one simple medicine at a time and in the least amount necessary. This is good science and common sense.

PLACEBO

This is an 'inactive' drug or sham treatment given to placate or 'please' the patient. The patient trusts the practitioner and believes that an active or genuine drug or treatment has been given. Orthodox medical thinking suggests that this belief may induce a psychosomatic benefit within the patient. How this happens is not understood and the placebo effect remains something of a mystery. (Ironically in the Randomised Controlled Trial (see 'Evidence') placebo is supposed to represent the known. It is the 'blank' or baseline against which active drugs and treatments are tested. This is clearly not a safe assumption.)

Any medical practitioner, of any kind, who does not acknowledge the potential power of placebo is a fool. It has been observed for centuries. To suggest that homoeopathic medicine works purely because of the placebo effect is also foolish. A scenario commonly encountered in homoeopathic medical practice makes my point:

A man develops a health problem. Sooner or later he takes his problem to his GP for diagnosis and treatment. Like most people in twenty-first century Western culture he has an inherent belief that this is the best, indeed only, course of action. He has started out with the belief that 'scientific medicine' will cure him. He has no reason to doubt this.

After several diagnoses, several visits to a consultant, and maybe half a dozen prescriptions of variously coloured 'state of the art' drugs (it is well known that coloured capsules induce a greater placebo response than white tablets) he is no better. He begins to feel disillusioned. He says things like 'I can't believe that in this day and age they can't find out what's wrong and sort me out!' His belief in 'scientific medicine' has been undermined, usually over quite some time because it was a strong belief. In desperation he visits a homoeopath and, after an hour or so of conversation, is given a single plain white tablet. The measure of his faith in the treatment is expressed through his exclamation: 'Is that it?'

Reluctantly, yet still desperate for relief, he decides to 'give it a go'. On his follow-up visit he declares that nothing has changed: 'I am no better'. After yet another conversation the homoeopath agrees that nothing has changed and decides, on the basis of some further information elicited from the patient, to prescribe a different plain white tablet. The patient agrees to give it 'one last shot'.

Two weeks later he calls to say 'I don't know what you gave me this time but my symptoms got a little worse for a few days and have now all gone. I can't believe it!' His improvement is apparently due to the placebo effect. Doesn't make a great deal of sense, does it?

It seems to me that the GP had the best chance to make use of the placebo effect, the consultant the next best chance and the homoeopath the least. And the frequently observed reaction of babies, unconscious people and animals (8) to homoeopathic medicines is unlikely to be due to any placebo effect either.

For over 200 years medical orthodoxy has dismissed the curative effects of homoeopathy as being due to 'mere placebo', 'just placebo', 'only placebo'. Three things are striking here:

1 If a patient cures him/herself because of their belief in the practitioner or treatment then there is clearly a profound connection between mind and body, psyche and soma. There are no molecules of 'active ingredient' involved.
2 To belittle this connection, this innate ability of a person to heal himself or herself, suggests arrogance.
3 To not invest time and money into the investigation of such ability for self-healing suggests negligence.

To dismiss the ability of humans to heal themselves through any means other than pharmaceutical drugs is disrespectful. It is incorrect, a delusion.

EVIDENCE

We need to know that a particular drug, medicine or treatment is both safe and effective if we are to use it with confidence. The current trend for 'evidence-based medicine' is relatively new and, rather alarmingly, early research in this field suggests that a large proportion of current medical practice has never been properly tested for effectiveness. In fact just 30 to 50% of medical practice in the UK today is supported by high-quality scientific evidence (9). This is not what we have been led to believe.

This also raises serious questions about why mainstream medicine is presented as being scientific, especially when homoeopathy is so heavily criticised for not being so. This strikes me as being hypocritical.

The 'gold standard' of clinical research is supposed to be the Randomised Controlled Trial (RCT), even though recent research suggests that the methodology of these studies is unrealistic and unscientific (10). Because homoeopathic treatment is individual and process orientated, taking place over time and sometimes involving the prescription of several medicines in sequence, it seems too complex a medical intervention to be explored through the methodology of the RCT. Good scientists are currently working to find a more appropriate methodology to test homoeopathy. Nevertheless, over 200 well-verified clinical trials and at least 5 meta-analyses of such trials have demonstrated the clinical effectiveness of homoeopathy (11). This evidence is generally ignored.

During the London cholera epidemic of 1854 the London Homoeopathic Hospital reported a fatality rate of 16.4%. The neighbouring
Middlesex Hospital reported a fatality rate of 53.2%. This evidence
was ignored too.

In September 2005 the Bristol Homoeopathic Hospital published the
results of a survey carried out by three of its doctors. Over a six-year
period, 6,544 consecutive patients, all with long-standing chronic
diseases such as asthma, migraine, IBS, arthritis, depression and chronic
fatigue syndrome, were treated homoeopathically. Seventy percent
of patients reported significant improvement in their condition and
51% felt much better (12). The media were informed of this but
were not interested.

In 2001 my own homoeopathic practice carried out an independent
audit. Again, 70% of patients reported 'significant improvement' in
their condition and 100% rated the care provided as 'excellent'.

Over 200 years, and in many countries, hundreds of millions of people
who are not stupid or easily fooled have found benefit through
homoeopathic treatment. I am not suggesting that such anecdotal
evidence is absolute proof that homoeopathy is effective; what I am
suggesting is that there might be something worthy of serious research.

Good science can be open-minded. Indeed open-mindedness is a prerequisite of good science. Until it is clearly understood how homoeopathy works, orthodox medical thinking will remain completely closed to the idea that it does work. The thought process: 'can't work therefore doesn't work...and is harmful', is poor science.

You may have come across research stories that 'prove beyond all doubt that homoeopathy is nonsense'. Many of these are simply stories. An example is the well-publicised RCT carried out at Exeter University into the effectiveness of Arnica (13). A key requirement of any RCT is that it must accurately reflect what actually happens in practice. This trial did not. I do not know one well-trained, experienced homoeopath who would prescribe in the way that the research indicated: this invalidates the experiment.

The main difficulty of doing serious research into homoeopathic medicine is lack of funds. Most homoeopaths are independent, free-thinking and ethical business people with not much free time or money. We have no back up and no government-funded research facilities. The major sponsor of medical research is the pharmaceutical industry and this is not likely to want to research a system of medicine that it cannot patent and make money from.

There is *enough evidence* for any sane and unprejudiced enquirer to show that homoeopathic treatment can be effective. Let's move on.

SAFETY

Homoeopathy was developed in response to the dangerous medical practices existing in the eighteenth century. It is one of the safest forms of medicine, even for babies, pregnant women and the elderly. Following treatment with a well-chosen medicine most people begin to feel better; for some people nothing happens. A small number of people experience some slight and temporary intensification of symptoms before they begin to improve.

Every year in the UK hundreds of thousands of people have their health undermined or destroyed as a direct result of mainstream medical intervention.

There is no comparison!

'As to diseases, make a habit of two things - to help or, at least, do no harm.'

Hippocrates

ETHICS

Most homoeopathic practices are independent and ethical small businesses. Most homoeopaths are registered with a professional organisation, adhere to a Code of Ethics, and go about their work quietly; making no great claims for what they achieve they let their results speak for themselves.

Big money is not being made, big advertising campaigns are not being mounted and fear is not being foisted upon the public.

The same cannot be said of the international pharmaceutical industry, the engine of mainstream medicine. This is inextricably linked to the petrochemical industry and world banking institutions and the only health with which it is concerned is healthy profit. A vast amount of money is being made.

Conventional drugs are becoming ever more expensive and increasing numbers of them are unaffordable even by the NHS in Britain. A recent study by the Office of Fair Trading (14) has revealed that the NHS is being grossly overcharged for drugs to the tune of £500 million. That is our money!

Drug companies spend huge amounts of money and use vast quantities of natural resources in developing, producing, packaging and selling their products, mainly to the 'developed' countries that can afford them.

Drug development involves testing powerful chemical agents on animals. This is both unethical and unscientific. Rats and rabbits are noticeably different to humans and disastrous consequences often arise when a drug under trial is given to people.

Many drugs are literally pushed onto the market, and alarming numbers are then withdrawn because they are not nearly as 'safe' as we were led to believe. From Thalidomide to Seroxat the same story is repeated over and over. It is simply not possible to predict the long-term effects of any drug: whilst humans have been around for hundreds of thousands of years, synthetic antibiotics, steroids, anti-depressants, contraceptive drugs etc. are new to planet Earth. In this sense at least, mainstream medical practice is experimental biology.

For the international pharmaceutical industry to continue to make huge amounts of money, humans have to continue to suffer. In fact, human suffering has to increase. This is especially the case for humans who can afford to pay.

Even within the medical establishment it is acknowledged that the drug industry is both under-regulated and overly powerful, controlling most medical research and publishing (15). Astonishingly, drug companies are allowed to evaluate their own products! This means that they can tell us a drug is safe when it is not. The current 'Seroxat' and 'Vioxx' scandals are likely to represent just the tip of a mighty iceberg, and many sources suggest that bribery and corruption are rampant in the international pharmaceutical industry.

This is not ethical business.

ECOLOGY

Homoeopathic pharmacies do not use chemical processes in the pro-duction of their medicines. Anything in nature is a potential medicine yet very little of it is needed in the preparation of a homoeopathic potency: the use of natural resources is kept to a minimum and the medicines produced are inexpensive, of high quality, effective for many years and harmless to the environment when disposed of correctly.

Orthodox medical drugs are produced through industrial processes that are not environmentally friendly. Synthetic purification and extraction processes are complex and solvent use is widespread. Drugs are researched, produced and packaged in huge quantities at great cost to both user and environment. Relative to homoeopathy the carbon footprint of mainstream medicine upon our planet has to be huge. The disposal of out of date, or 'unsafe', drugs and chemicals takes place through dumping: dumping in the earth; dumping in the sky (through incineration); dumping in Third World nations. Dumping is likely to have a profound impact upon the environment.

From a global perspective we are just beginning to discover the potential impact on our environment of the large-scale production and widespread and indiscriminate use of antibiotics.

The biosphere on this planet is essentially bacterial. Bacteria are the most successful organisms in the history of life on Earth. They are everywhere, from frozen seas to burning deserts to hospital operating theatres. Ninety percent of the cells in your body space are microbial, i.e. bacteria, viruses and fungi (16). Ninety-seven percent of all bacteria are either harmless or helpful to humans. As an example, the twenty trillion in your gut at this moment are helping you by producing essential vitamins and protecting you from the bacteria that could cause harm.

Bacteria have helped to shape the environment. Wherever there is life there will be death - and bacteria, breaking down organic matter in endless cycles of growth and decay. They are the great recyclers, constantly maintaining the integrity of life on Earth, the biosphere.

And we have flooded this vibrant biosphere with 'anti-bio' agents. We have created a huge number of antibiotics and antiseptics and have used them to excess in humans and animals. We have upset the natural balance on many levels in our indiscriminate attempts to conquer and destroy. In doing so we have undermined our health and helped create the 'Superbug': antibiotic resistance is now posing a serious threat, particularly with regard to MRSA infections and diseases like tuberculosis which were once considered 'defeated'.

The arrogance of a medical establishment that has believed it could dominate the natural world and eradicate infectious disease, and has boasted of the antibiotic as its proudest achievement, is extraordinary.

When medicine is practised with both art and science, when true healing takes place, then humility is always present.

EQUALITY

All people regardless of age, gender, race or creed can benefit from homoeopathic treatment. Even sceptics!

Babies and children benefit markedly from treatment started early on in life. Our senior citizens too can be helped to improve their quality of life. Many of them feel that doctors discriminate against patients over the age of 65 and give them less time, poorer advice and worse treatment than younger people.

Homoeopaths do not discriminate against anybody and respect and give time to the elders in their communities.

Based as it is on pure observation and experience, homoeopathy can bring benefit without any compromise of religious belief. You do not have to believe in homoeopathy but you may want to give it a chance.

THE CONSULTATION

The homoeopathic consultation is a unique experience in medicine. You will very rarely have the opportunity to be listened to with such close attention. There are few other situations in which your health and yourself are explored so thoroughly.

This can be a very empowering experience. To move toward an understanding of yourself and your health within the context of your life can enable you to regain perspective and engage in a process of self-healing and discovery.

This kind of consultation is one of the high arts of medicine and needs to be experienced to be appreciated.

As well as exploring your current complaint(s) in great detail, the homoeopath will gather information about YOU. 'You are what you eat' may have some truth in it but 'you are what you think and feel' has much deeper resonance with your life and health. Together you will explore your reactions to your environment, other people, stress, food etc. Your sleep, dream and hormonal patterns will be looked into as well as your personal and family medical history.

It can be difficult, with so much information, to find an individual prescription for you so you are encouraged to be as clear as you can about any information you give. It is also very helpful to the homoeopath if you have thought about these things before your visit.

CONTINUING TREATMENT

It is not always possible to obtain all the information needed for an accurate prescription in just one visit. It may be necessary to engage in several consultations before you and your complaint can be fully understood. In fact homoeopathic treatment rarely involves a one-off meeting. It is a collaborative process that takes place over time and through a number of consultations.

It usually takes time for you to develop any given complaint and so it makes sense that it will take some time to return to good health. If you have been taking a number of drugs prescribed by your doctor for some time then this can slow down your response to homoeopathic treatment. Be patient.

Often the changes that follow your first prescription necessitate another different medicine to be prescribed. Cure is not a one-off event, it is a process that you are encouraged to fully participate in.

'It is not enough for (the doctor) to do what (he) can do; the patient and his environment have to contribute to achieve a cure.'

Hippocrates

Once you have returned to health the focus of treatment changes. Keeping well means continuing to pay attention to your health. It may involve dealing with any tendencies to ill health that are part of your basic nature. This is called 'constitutional treatment' and it has been shown to be effective in sustaining and nourishing health and wellbeing.

If you have joined a recognised homoeopathic practice then you have a resource for any health issues in the future. A good homoeopath knows that a homoeopathic approach is not always the best one in all circumstances and will often be able to refer you to another kind of practitioner, one more appropriate to your needs. These practitioners may include a GP, an osteopath, a psychotherapist, acupuncturist etc.

RECOMMENDATIONS

Recommendations are the life-blood of homoeopathic practice. Ninety-nine percent of people who consult with me have been recommended by other people, people who have benefited from my treatment. People come because they have tried everything that mainstream medicine has to offer and are no better. They hear of someone they trust or respect having been helped by homoeopathy and they pick up the phone.

They have not come as the result of persuasive advertising that offers 'miracle cures' or false hopes.

To be recommended means that I must have helped someone with his or her health problems. I must have met some needs that were not being met by mainstream medicine.

I have to be good at what I do and I have to keep working at being as good as I can be. People pay me to help them, and my 'competition', i.e. the NHS, is said to be 'free' (of course this is not actually true because we pay for the services through taxation). If I don't help people then word gets around and I go out of business. It's that simple.

I have been practising and earning a modest living for myself and my family for over 15 years and this simple fact tells me I am doing something useful that many people value.

Interestingly, a GP does not have to be any good as a practitioner, does not have to get good results. I wonder how busy GPs might be if we all had to pay for treatment?

TIME

The amount of time given to consultation varies from practitioner to practitioner. An initial consultation generally lasts around an hour and a half, whilst follow-up appointments take 30 minutes to one hour. Appointments for children tend to take less time: around one hour and 30 minutes respectively. This is quite different to the 6-10 minutes allowed by a GP.

'How many times will I have to come and see you?' is clearly a good question. Equally clearly, it is not possible to say for sure. You are an individual and your process of cure is individual. Generally it might be said that the longer you have been unwell the longer you will take to get well.

If you are not willing to give time to your process of becoming well again then you are less likely to get well and are more likely to become un-well again. As a culture we do not allow enough time for recovery, convalescence or rest. Time really can be a great healer, if we allow it.

MONEY

The fee charged for an adult's initial consultation is generally between £40 and £90, with follow-up consultations costing £30-£45. The fee charged for a child's initial consultation is around £30-£60, and £20-£40 for a follow-up. These fees usually include the cost of the medicines.

Some people think that this is expensive.

If you were to consult privately with an orthodox doctor you would expect to pay a lot more. It is not uncommon to be charged between £90-£160 for a half-hour appointment. This does not usually include any treatments or drugs.

There is no comparison.

Most of us who live in twenty-first century Britain can afford to consult with a homoeopath. We spend a lot of money on food, clothing, cars and leisure. It is simply a question of priority. Perhaps because health care in this country has been free for so long we are just not inclined to pay for it. Or value it.

For most of us it is a matter of choice. How much time and money are you willing to invest in your health and that of your family?

So, homoeopathic treatment is relatively inexpensive. Furthermore, successful homoeopathic treatment can save the NHS a lot of money, money that could be better used on other aspects of our health.

THE NATIONAL HEALTH SERVICE

It is a little known fact that patients in England and Wales have the right to request homoeopathic treatment through the NHS. This will usually involve a referral to their nearest homoeopathic hospital; these are located in London, Tunbridge Wells, Liverpool and Bristol (there is also one in Glasgow).

The Royal London Homoeopathic Hospital handles over 30,000 patient appointments every year, and most of these patients are referred by their GPs (17). Presumably the GPs referred because they were not able to help with mainstream medical treatment and thought their patients would benefit from the homoeopathic approach.

The RLHH remains one of the very few NHS establishments not making a huge financial loss whilst providing a service that is greatly appreciated by patients. Nevertheless, critics of homoeopathy want this hospital closed down so that funding can be used for 'more useful and necessary medical research and treatments'.

How much funding is involved? The NHS currently spends around £5.5 million a year on homoeopathic hospitals in England and contributed towards the £20 million cost of refurbishing the RLHH (18). It also spends £27 million a day on drugs that we habitually use and wastes £200 million every year on drugs that are never used (19). Furthermore, around £500 million could be saved each year if the pharmaceutical industry sold drugs to the NHS for a fair price (14).

In the face of such massive expenditure the argument to close the homoeopathic hospitals to save money becomes absurd.

The NHS spends billions of pounds on medical research and treatment every year yet disease continues to spiral out of control. Everywhere we read that 'the NHS is in melt-down', overwhelmed by increasing numbers of patients and increasing costs. At the same time, around 470,000 people privately consult with a homoeopath each year (20), representing a significant saving to the NHS and a clear demand for this form of treatment. It seems increasingly obvious that the health of the nation would best be served by an integrated approach to medicine, with all of us working together.

DOCTORS

*'The physician's highest and only calling is to make
the sick healthy, to cure, as it is called.'*

Dr S. Hahnemann, Founder of Homoeopathy

Most people do not realise that hundreds of thousands of fully trained doctors, in many parts of the world, also practise homoeopathic medicine. Generally, these doctors have been independent-thinking enough to seriously question what they were doing and why they were doing it. These doctors have noticed that chronic diseases are increasing and that people are suffering as a direct result of the drugs and treatments they have been prescribed. These doctors have not been content to continue to do harm and have searched for other less damaging ways to help their patients.

This is following in the tradition of Dr. Samuel Hahnemann (1755-1843), the physician responsible for formulating homoeopathy into the system of medicine we practise today. Dismayed at the damage he was causing to his patients he stopped practising medicine and earned much less of a living for himself and his family by translating medical textbooks. Whilst doing this he famously questioned that Cinchona bark was the cure for malaria 'because of its bitter effect upon the stomach'. He decided to take some of this drug himself and discovered that it induced in him all the symptoms of malaria. This was when he began to wonder about the idea that 'like cures like'.

Fluent in English, French, Italian, Greek, Latin and Hebrew, Hahnemann rigorously applied scientific methodology to his investigations of what must have seemed at the time a new world of biology and medicine.

In the cholera epidemic of 1854 a Dr. Macloughlin was appointed medical inspector to observe the progress of the disease at the London Homoeopathic Hospital. He was an orthodox practitioner, an expert in cholera and a self-confessed enemy of the 'homoeopathic system'. All the same, he concluded that if he were to be stricken by cholera he 'would rather be in the hands of a homoeopathic than an allopathic (orthodox) advisor' (21). This is a very common story.

Professor Jacques Benveniste, a doctor and allergy specialist, was research director at the French National Institute for Health and Medical Research during the 1980's. In 1985 one of his research assistants found some results that made no sense: a solution that had accidentally been diluted to the point where there was no possibility of any molecule remaining was found to have a biological effect. Benveniste, who had not even heard of homoeopathy, dismissed the result as an error but asked the technician to repeat the experiment. The same results were obtained.

Benveniste was a well-respected establishment scientist who came across something he could not explain...but he did not ignore it or cover it up. He pursued his research and produced sound and reproducible data demonstrating the biological effect of high dilutions. He coined the term 'the memory of water' to describe a possible mechanism for what he observed. Nature magazine, a prestigious scientific publication, infamously sent a team to investigate - a team made up of a journalist, a writer on fraud and a magician.

Benveniste became the focus of a scientific witch hunt. His work was dismissed as a 'delusion', his professional competence, mental balance and scientific integrity questioned and his impressive reputation destroyed...by prejudice and poor science (22).

Hahnemann, Macloughlin, Benveniste and many other doctors and scientists, even today, have been ridiculed and reviled for their support of homoeopathic medicine. It seems extraordinary to think that well-qualified and experienced doctors and scientists are likely to be charmed into a 'system of quackery' without being significantly impressed by its effectiveness. This is especially so if we consider the social, economic and professional losses they would have incurred.

VOCATION

People do not train to become homoeopathic medical practitioners for money or prestige. Most have been so impressed by a personal experience of homoeopathy that they want to study it and be able to offer it to others.

A properly qualified homoeopath will have studied hard for at least 3-4 years, to degree level or higher. He/she will have paid for that basic training themselves because there are no grants available at this time. Once licensed to practice she/he has to find the money to set up in business, to pay for clinic space and insurance, and buy all necessary equipment, books and medicines.

To register with a professional organisation requires a significant annual subscription. Continuing professional development is a requirement of registration and also has to be paid for by the homoeopath.

The financial reward for a successful homoeopath is around a quarter of the salary of a GP.

In addition to working hard to deserve the privilege of being asked to help you, the homoeopath is frequently subjected to, generally unfounded yet still annoying, ridicule and derision from orthodox medicine and the press. Whilst this may be character strengthening it is also tedious and wearisome!

Any homoeopath you may visit has committed, and continues to commit, a great deal of themselves to their work.

Just as there are bogus doctors so there are bogus homoeopaths and you are strongly advised to only approach a fully qualified and registered practitioner.

HOPE

Critics of homoeopathy have often charged homoeopaths with offering 'false hope' to people. This is not true.

Homoeopathy has produced some marvellous results during the last 200 years yet it cannot cure everything. Of course it cannot because it is a system of medicine not a source of miracles. Since every person is an individual there is always hope, even in palliative care of the terminally ill, for some improvement in health and quality of life.

Hope is not the same as false hope; but hope can make all the difference to an outcome.

END

I am sure that we would all agree with Hippocrates: 'As to diseases, make a habit of two things - to help or, at least, do no harm'. And with Hahnemann: 'The highest ideal of cure is the rapid, gentle and permanent restoration of health...'

Homoeopathic medicine offers safe, effective, inexpensive, ethical and environmentally friendly solutions to health problems of all kinds. Millions of people will testify to this truth.

Many people who try homoeopathic treatment have tried everything that mainstream medicine has to offer and are no better. Around 70% of people experience significant improvement in their symptoms or health as a result of homoeopathic treatment. If such an improvement is purely due to the placebo effect and talking with the homoeopath then homoeopaths are clearly very gifted listeners!

When sound evidence exists to support homoeopathy and there is no evidence that it does any harm then why is it subjected to such hostile criticism by the orthodox medical establishment?

'All truth passes through three stages.
First, it is ridiculed.
Second, it is violently opposed.
Third, it is accepted as self-evident.'

Schopenhauer

REFERENCES

1   Matthews, R. (2006). The Quantum Elixir. *New Scientist*, 8 April.

2   Hitchen, L. (2006). Adverse Drug Reactions Result in 250,000 UK Hospital Admissions a Year. *British Medical Journal* 332(7550):1109.

3   Henry, R.C. (2006). The Mental Universe. *Nature* 436:29.

4   Gascoigne, S. (2003). *The Prescribed Drugs Guide – A Holistic Perspective*. Jigme Press.

5   Macdonald, M. (1998). Thousands in Worse Health After Hospital. *The Telegraph*, 8 November.

6   Null, G.N., Dean, C., Feldman, M., Rasio, D. & Smith, D. (2004). Death by Medicine: an Independent Review Commissioned by the Nutrition Institute of America. Life Extension Foundation, www.lef.org/magazine/mag2006/aug2006_report_death_01.htm.

7   Pert, C.B. (1998). *Molecules of Emotion - Why You Feel the Way You Feel*. Simon & Schuster UK Ltd.

8   Hektoen, L. (2005). Review of the Current Involvement of Homeopathy in Veterinary Practice and Research. *The Veterinary Record* 157(8): 224-9.

9   Shaw, S. (2006). A Critical Approach to Evidence Provided Through Clinical Trials. *Nursing Times* 102(36): 36-8.

10 Penston, J. (2005). Large Scale Randomised Trials - a Misguided Approach to Clinical Research. *Medical Hypotheses* 64(3): 651-7.

11 Reilly, D. (2005). Homeopathy: Increasing Scientific Validation. *Alternative Therapies* 11(2): 31.

12 Spence, D.S., Thompson, E.A. & Baron, S.J. (2005). Homeopathic Treatment for Chronic Disease: a Six-Year University-Hospital Outpatient Observational Study. *Journal of Alternative and Complementary Medicine* 11(5): 793-8.

13 Stevinson, C., Devaraj, V.S., Fountain-Barber, A., Hawkins, S. & Ernst, E. (2003). Homeopathic Arnica for Prevention of Pain and Bruising: Randomised Placebo-Controlled Trial in Hand Surgery. *Journal of the Royal Society of Medicine* 96: 60-5.

14 Office of Fair Trading website: www.oft.gov.uk/news/press/2007/29-07

15 Godlee, F. (2006). Can We Tame the Monster? *British Medical Journal* 333(7558): 53.

16 Vermeulen, F. (2005). *Monera: Kingdom Bacteria and Viruses.* Emryss Publishers, Haarlem, The Netherlands.

17 University College London Hospitals website: www.uclh.nhs.uk/RLHH.

18 Campbell, D. & Fitzgerald, M. (2007). The Queen Loves it, but Royals' Favoured Hospital Faces Closure. *The Observer*, 8 April.

19 Lakhani, N. (2007). Pharmageddon. *The Independent*, 26 August.

20 Society of Homoeopaths website: www.homeopathy-soh.org.

21 www.homeoint.org/morrell/british/evidence.htm

22 Schiff, M. (1995). *The Memory of Water: Homoeopathy and the Battle of New Ideas in the New Science.* Thorsons, London.

RESOURCES

Books

Capra, F. (1983). *The Tao of Physics*. Flamingo, London.

Castro, M. (1990). *The Complete Homeopathy Handbook*. Macmillan London Ltd.

Coulter, H.L. (1981). *Homoeopathic Science and Modern Medicine*. North Atlantic Books.

Coulter, H.L. (1990). *Vaccination, Social Violence and Criminality*. North Atlantic Books.

Gunn, T. (1992). *Mass Vaccination: A Point in Question*. Cutting Edge Publications, Cumbria.

Gunn, T. (2006). *Comparing Natural Immunity with Vaccination*. The Informed Parent Publications, West Sussex.

Hahnemann, S. *Organon of the Medical Art* (edited and annotated by Wenda Brewster O'Reilly and based on a translation by Steven Decker: adapted from the sixth edition of the *Organon der Heilkunst* completed by Samuel Hahnemann in 1842). Birdcage Books, Redmond, Washington,1996.

Le Fanu, J. (2000). *The Rise & Fall of Modern Medicine*. Abacus, London.

McTaggart, L. (1996). *What Doctors Don't Tell You: The Truth About the Dangers of Modern Medicine*. Thorsons, London.

McTaggart, L. (2001). *The Field - The Quest for the Secret Force of the Universe*. HarperCollins Publishers Ltd.

Mendelson, R.S. (1979). *Confessions of a Medical Heretic*. Contemporary Books, Chicago.

Morrish, M. (2006). *Medicine Flows - Homoeopathic Philosophy*. The Homeopathy Centre, Bristol.

Vithoulkas, G. (1991). *A New Model for Health and Disease*. Health and Habitat and North Atlantic Books.

Papers

Chyka, P.A. (2000). How Many Deaths Occur Annually from Adverse Drug Reactions in the United States? *American Journal of Medicine* 109(2):122-30.

Colloca, C. & Benedetti, F. (2005). Placebo and Painkillers: Is Mind as Real as Matter? *Nature Reviews Neurosciences* 6:545-52.

Connor, S. (2004). Sceptic's Tests Support Homoeopathy. *The Independent*, 19 August.

Dixon, D.M., Sweeney, K.G. & Perreira Gray, D.J. (1999). The Physician Healer: Ancient Magic or Modern Science? *British Journal of General Practice*, 49:309-12.

Kaptchuk, T.J. (2001). The Double-Blind, Randomised, Placebo-Controlled Trial: Gold Standard or Golden Calf? *Journal of Clinical Epidemiology* 54:541-9.

Lazarou, J., Pomeranz, B.H. & Corey, P.N. (1998). Incidence of Adverse Drug Reactions in Hospitalised Patients: A Meta-Analysis of Prospective Studies. *Journal of the American Medical Association* 279:1200-5.

Linde, K., Clausius, N., Ramirez, G. (1997). Are the Clinical Effects of Homoeopathy Placebo Effects? A Meta-Analysis of Placebo-Controlled Trials. *Lancet* 350:834-43.

Mastrangelo, D. (2005). The Growth of a Lie and the End of 'Conventional' Medicine. *Medical Sciences Monitor* 11(12):27-31.

Mastrangelo, D. (2007). Hormesis, Epitaxy, the Structure of Liquid Water and the Science of Homeopathy. *Homeopathy in Practice: Summer ed.*

Reilly D., Taylor, M.A. & Beattie, N.G.M. (1994). Is Evidence for Homeopathy Reproducible? *Lancet* 344:1601-6.

Weatherley-Jones, E., Thompson, E.A. & Thomas, K.J. (2004). The Placebo-Controlled Trial as a Test of Complementary and Alternative Medicine: Observations from Research Experience of Individualised Homeopathic Treatment. *Homeopathy* 93:186-189.

Organisations
Society of Homeopaths
0845 450 6611
www.homeopathy-soh.org

Homeopathic Medical Association
01474 560 336
www.the-hma.org

Alliance of Registered Homeopaths
0870 073 6339
www.a-r-h.org

British Homeopathic Association
0870 444 3950
www.trusthomeopathy.org

National Institute for Health and
Clinical Excellence
www.nice.org.uk

Education
Homeopathy Course Providers Forum
01444 236 848
www.hcpf.org.uk

Bookshops
Alternative Training
0800 0439 349
www.alternative-training.com

Minerva
01225 760 003
www.minervabooks.co.uk

The Homeopathic Book Company
01476 550 754
www.homeopathicbooks.co.uk

Homoeopathic Pharmacies
Helios Homoeopathy
01892 537254
www.helios.co.uk

Ainsworths
0207 7935 5330
www.ainsworths.com

Nelsons Homeopathic Pharmacy
0207 629 3118
www.nelsonshp.com

ABOUT THE AUTHOR

I am a scientist by training and a fully qualified and registered homoeopath. I have been practising homoeopathic medicine for over 15 years
and I believe this has helped me to become a more rounded natural
scientist. I do not profess to be an expert in any field, I simply spend my
working life helping others to find solutions to their health problems.

This is similar to the work of doctors and a whole legion of healthcare
practitioners - I simply bring a different approach to that work.

To be clear: I have enormous respect and admiration for those
doctors, nurses and healthcare practitioners who devote their time
and energy to helping us. I have no respect for cynicism, arrogance,
fear-mongering, fraud, ill logic or poor science in medicine.

I am wary of any medical approach that is not based upon sound
principles and very suspicious of a pharmaceutical industry that seems
to lack moral principles.

It is clear to me that disease continues to increase on planet Earth and
that no one system of medicine has a monopoly on getting people
better. It is also clear to me that the only sane solution is for us all to
work together in an integrated manner.

It is my experience that a lot of people feel the same way.